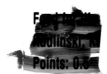

Science Links

Food for Life

Kathleen V. Kudlinski

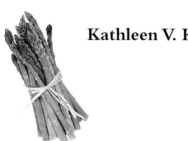
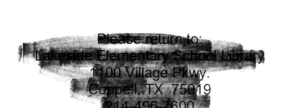

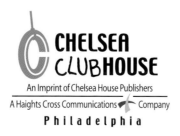

CHELSEA CLUBHOUSE

An Imprint of Chelsea House Publishers

A Haights Cross Communications Company

Philadelphia

This edition first published in 2003 by Chelsea Clubhouse, a division of
Chelsea House Publishers and a subsidiary of Haights Cross Communications.

A Haights Cross Communications Company

This edition was adapted from Newbridge Discovery Links® by arrangement with Newbridge Educational Publishing.
All rights reserved. No part of this publication may be reproduced or transmitted in any form or by any means without
the written permission of the publisher. Printed and bound in the United States of America.

Chelsea Clubhouse
1974 Sproul Road, Suite 400
Broomall, PA 19008-0914

The Chelsea House world wide web address is www.chelseahouse.com

Library of Congress Cataloging-in-Publication Data
Kudlinski, Kathleen V.
   Food for life / by Kathleen V. Kudlinski.
      v. cm. — (Science links)
Includes index.
Contents: Sipping sugar — Raccoons' rules — Eating energy — Breakfast with the bats —
Clues from a camel.
   ISBN 0-7910-7421-8
   1. Nutrition—Juvenile literature. [1. Nutrition. 2. Food habits. 3. Animals—Food.] I. Title.
II. Series.
   QP141 .K797 2003
   613.2—dc21
                                                                                                      2002015889

Copyright © Newbridge Educational Publishing LLC

Newbridge Discovery Links Guided Reading Program Author: Dr. Brenda Parkes
Content Reviewers: Dr. Clifford Lo, Children's Hospital, Harvard Medical School, Boston, MA; Dr.
Ellen Dierenfeld, Wildlife Conservation Society, Bronx, NY
Written by Kathleen V. Kudlinski

Cover Photograph: Food groups on a fork
Table of Contents Photograph: Squirrel eating walnuts

Photo Credits:
Cover: Michael Mahovlich/Masterfile; Title page: CORBIS; Table of Contents page: Dianna Sarto/CorbisStockMarket;
page 4: M.P.L. Fogden/Bruce Coleman, Inc.; page 5: Charles Gupton/CorbisStockMarket; page 7: Mug
Shots/CorbisStockMarket; page 8: Gay Bumgarner; page 9: Gerhard Steiner/CorbisStockMarket; page 10: CORBIS;
page 11: T. & P. Leeson/Photo Researchers; page 12: George Shelley/CorbisStockMarket; page 13: Vittoriano
Rastelli/CORBIS; page 14: CORBIS; page 15: S. Dalton/Photo Researchers; page 16: Anthony Johnson/Image Bank;
page 17: Rita Maas/Image Bank; page 18: David Stoecklein/CorbisStockMarket; page 19: Guido Alberto Rossi/Image
Bank; page 20: Joseph Sohm/ChromoSohm/CORBIS; page 21: (top) Patrick Lacroix/Image Bank, (bottom) CORBIS;
page 22: CORBIS

Illustration on page 9 by Barb Cousins

While every care has been taken to trace and acknowledge photo copyrights for this edition, the publisher apologizes
for any accidental infringement where copyright has proved untraceable.

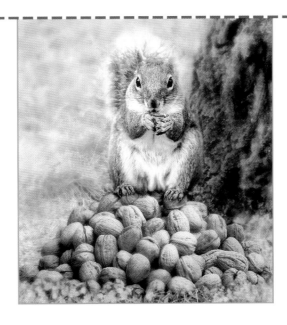

Table of Contents

Sipping Sugar

A nimals are great athletes. They run and leap, fly and climb, gallop and paddle. Where do they get all that energy? It comes from eating foods that are just right for their bodies.

  With their tiny bodies and long bills, hummingbirds are built to sip sweet nectar from flowers. But when scientists looked into hummingbirds' stomachs, they also found tiny spiders and flies. This showed scientists that hummingbirds need more than one kind of food to be healthy.

To flap its wings more than 50 times a second, this hummingbird needs all the energy it can get from feeding on nectar and insects.

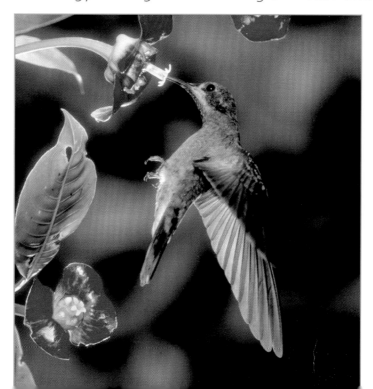

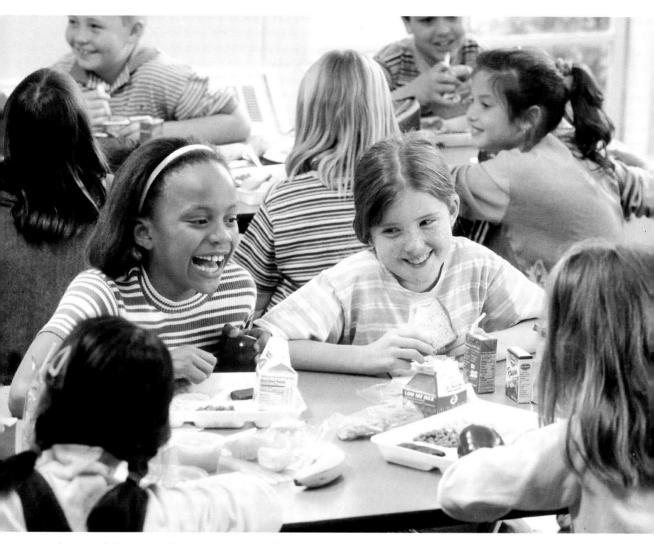

These children's hearts pump about 80 times every minute. That takes energy!

Your body, like that of the hummingbird, needs a mix of foods. To stay healthy, you need as many as 83 different chemical substances, called **nutrients**. It sounds complicated, but you don't have to keep track of all of them. Scientists have grouped the foods into a special chart. All you need to do is eat servings from each food group every day.

The chart is shaped like a pyramid. The foods on the bottom level are full of energy-storing nutrients called **carbohydrates**. Rice, corn, and wheat are carbohydrates. They can be made into flours that are used in breads, pasta, cereals, and tortillas. Potatoes and peas are also rich in carbohydrates.

Other foods from plants are on the next level. Plants are packed with **vitamins** that they make themselves. As they grow, plants also take in **minerals** from the ground. Eating fruits and vegetables is the best way to get these nutrients.

The **protein** foods come next. Your body has to have protein to grow and build strong muscles. Meat, chicken, and fish contain lots of protein. Dairy foods like milk and cheese provide protein plus calcium for strong bones and teeth.

Sugar, oil, and fats are at the top of the pyramid. You need just a little of these foods.

Why do you think the food chart is shaped like a pyramid?

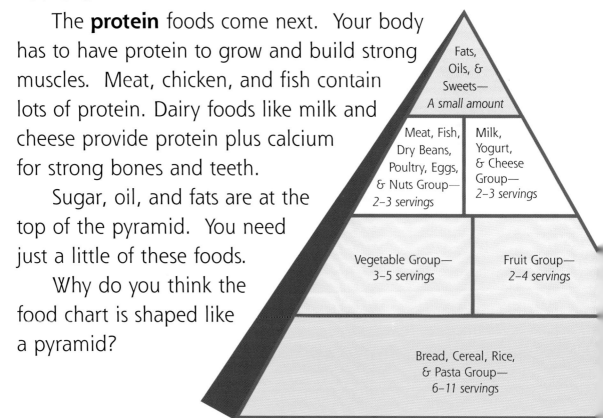

Fats, Oils, & Sweets— A small amount

Meat, Fish, Dry Beans, Poultry, Eggs, & Nuts Group— 2–3 servings

Milk, Yogurt, & Cheese Group— 2–3 servings

Vegetable Group— 3–5 servings

Fruit Group— 2–4 servings

Bread, Cereal, Rice, & Pasta Group— 6–11 servings

Recommended Dietary Guidelines issued by the U.S. Department of Agriculture and the U.S. Department of Health and Human Services

Can you match up the
foods in this pyramid
with those listed in the
chart on page 6?

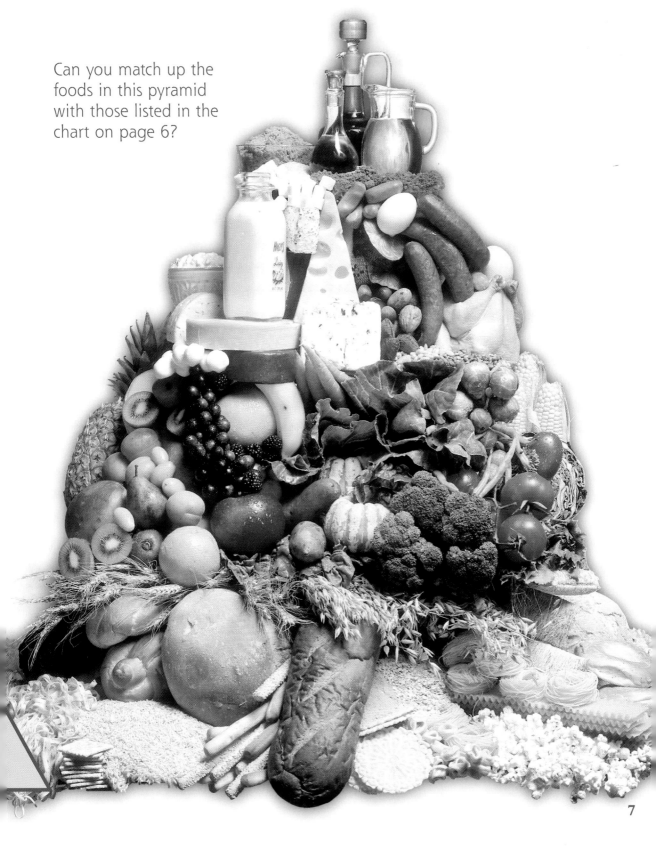

Raccoons' Rules

Mother raccoons teach their babies how to find lots of foods from the protein group: crayfish, bird's eggs, clams, and beetles. They eat plants, too: corn and seeds, nuts and mushrooms, fruits and berries, stems and juicy roots.

Scientists call animals like raccoons **omnivores** (from the Latin *omni*, which means "everything," and *vorare*, which means "to eat"). **Carnivores** (from *carne*, which means "meat") mainly eat meat. Plant-eaters are **herbivores**. Look back at the food pyramid. What kind of eater are you?

What foods might these baby raccoons find here?

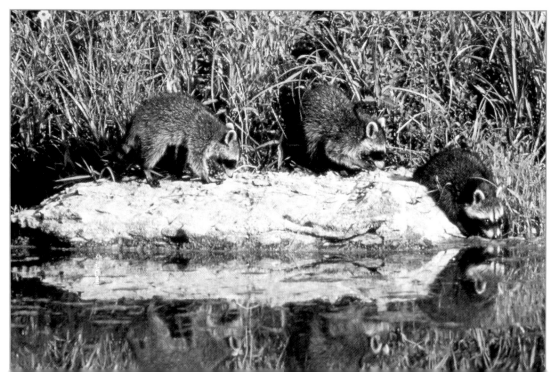

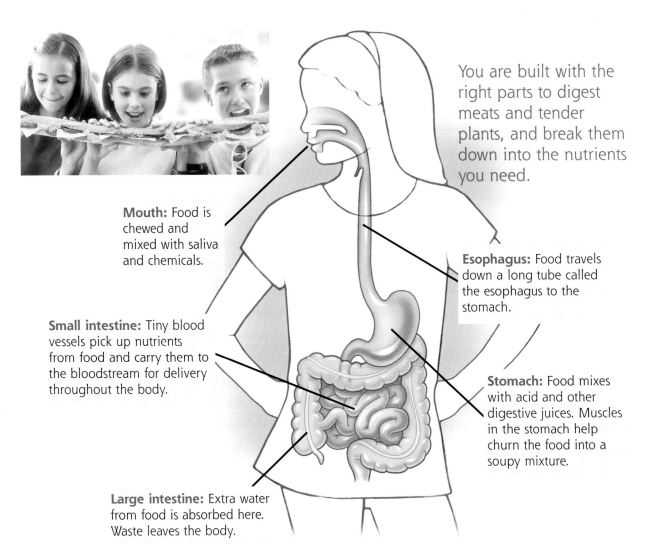

You are built with the right parts to digest meats and tender plants, and break them down into the nutrients you need.

Mouth: Food is chewed and mixed with saliva and chemicals.

Esophagus: Food travels down a long tube called the esophagus to the stomach.

Small intestine: Tiny blood vessels pick up nutrients from food and carry them to the bloodstream for delivery throughout the body.

Stomach: Food mixes with acid and other digestive juices. Muscles in the stomach help churn the food into a soupy mixture.

Large intestine: Extra water from food is absorbed here. Waste leaves the body.

Carnivores have a very simple system that enables them to **digest** their food easily. Like you, they chew their food and swallow it. Then the food travels to the stomach, the small intestine, and the large intestine.

It's harder to digest plants, so most herbivores are built differently. Cows eat mainly grass, but they need three extra compartments in their stomachs to digest this high-fiber **diet**.

"People food" offers lots of choices. This is a good thing. You wouldn't want to eat nothing but fish or chew on broccoli all day long.

You get the nutrients you need by eating a variety of foods within each group. Look at the vitamin chart below to see why. No one food has every vitamin.

But you don't need to carry around a chart to stay healthy. Just remember to eat like an omnivore!

Of all these vitamins, D is the only one your own body can make. To do that, you need to be in sunlight. Which foods supply more than one vitamin?

VITAMIN	BEST SOURCES	PARTS OF THE BODY IT HELPS
A	Sweet potatoes, carrots, broccoli, kale, cantaloupe	Eyes, skin. Helps fight diseases and heal cuts.
C	Oranges, lemons, grapefruit, cantaloupe, strawberries, broccoli, tomatoes, potatoes, brussels sprouts	Skin, teeth, bones. Helps heal wounds, fight infections, and mend broken bones.
D	Sunlight, milk, egg yolks	Teeth, bones
E	Spinach, carrots, celery, peanuts, vegetable oil, cabbage, broccoli	Blood, lungs
K	Green beans, tomatoes, cabbage, spinach, broccoli, lettuce	Helps heal cuts.

Your body also needs B vitamins. The most important vitamins from the B group are B_1, B_2, niacin, B_6, and B_{12}. These nutrients are found mainly in meat, fish, poultry, and grains, and they help the body by keeping the blood healthy, fighting disease, and turning food into energy.

Eating Energy

A deer has to chew plants all day long for energy. A wolf only needs one meaty meal to get the energy it needs. How can that be?

Some foods have more energy stored inside than others. Scientists measure this kind of energy as **calories**. Leaves are low in calories. A cup of lettuce has only around nine calories. Meat, especially fatty meat, is a high-calorie food. A quarter-pound cooked hamburger patty has around 300 calories. You can see that a mouthful of lettuce provides a lot less energy than a mouthful of meat.

Plants are the right food to give these deer the energy they need to zip through the grass.

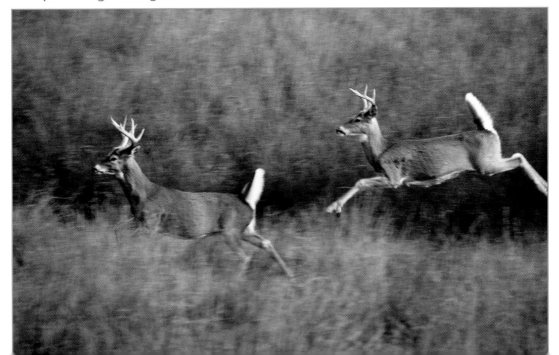

You need to eat around 2,000 calories every day. This gives you the energy to power your growing body, to breathe, to keep your heart and muscles strong, to stay warm, to heal from sickness or scrapes, to digest your food, and even to think. Men burn more calories than women, and everyone burns more when they are active.

Sometimes the numbers add up but the nutrients don't! For example, butter and sugar are high in calories. A lunch box full of candy bars holds more calories than you would

There are lots of ways to get a good workout.

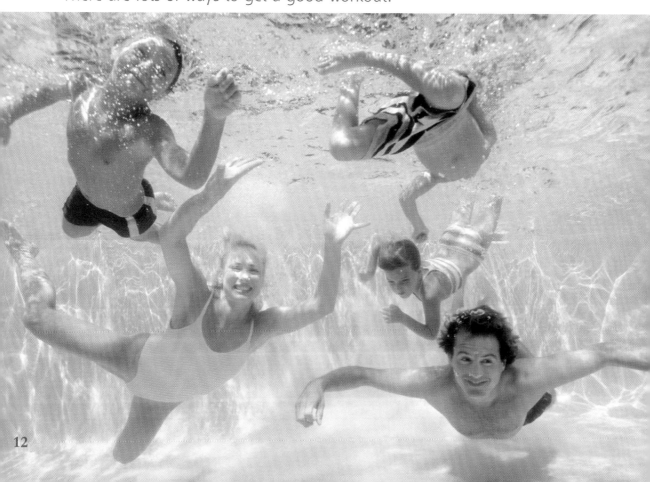

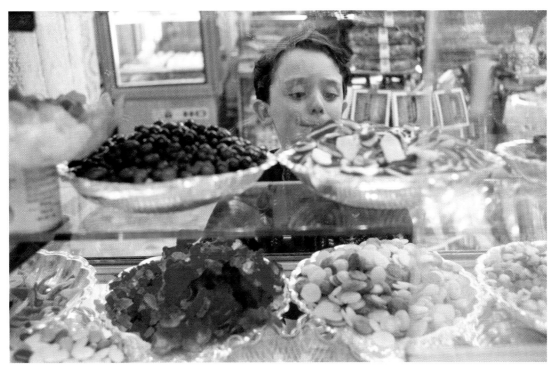

What nutrients do you think you would get from these foods?

need in a whole day. But there is a problem. Candy bars are low in valuable nutrients. After you eat them, your body is still hungry for the vitamins, minerals, and protein it needs. Also, those extra calories are stored as fat.

Fat isn't all bad. You need some fat to build brain cells, cushion your heart and other organs, and help maintain your body temperature. But storing too much fat can slow you down and make you sick.

Which foods will you choose to stay healthy and full of energy?

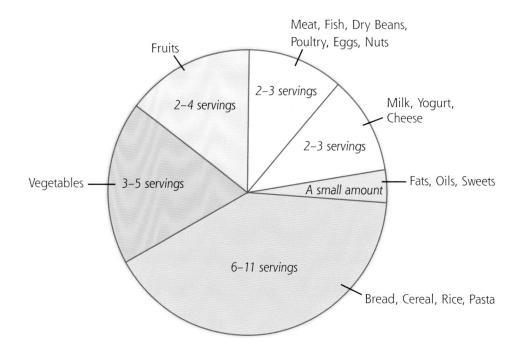

Fruits — 2–4 servings

Meat, Fish, Dry Beans, Poultry, Eggs, Nuts — 2–3 servings

Milk, Yogurt, Cheese — 2–3 servings

Fats, Oils, Sweets — A small amount

Vegetables — 3–5 servings

Bread, Cereal, Rice, Pasta — 6–11 servings

Food for a Day

Here's a menu for one day.

What foods could you add from the protein or carbohydrate groups to make the menu more complete? What foods could you substitute to make the menu more nutritious?

Use the information in the pie chart to help you.

Menu

Breakfast	cereal cantaloupe milk
Lunch	vegetable soup cheeseburger pear soda
Snack	cookies milk
Dinner	chicken baked potato broccoli ice cream milk
Snack	popcorn apple juice

Breakfast with the Bats

Most bats sleep all day long, burning energy just by staying alive. When they wake up at dusk, they need to replace those calories, and quickly.

To break their **fast**, or time without food, the bats swoop out from attics and caves, sip some water, and start hunting. Insect-eating bats catch up to 600 insects an hour.

After a night's sleep, you need a meal to break your fast, too.

There are calories in all foods, even the moths that bats eat. What would you call a bat's breakfast cereal? Moth Flakes? Mosquito Crispies? What else?

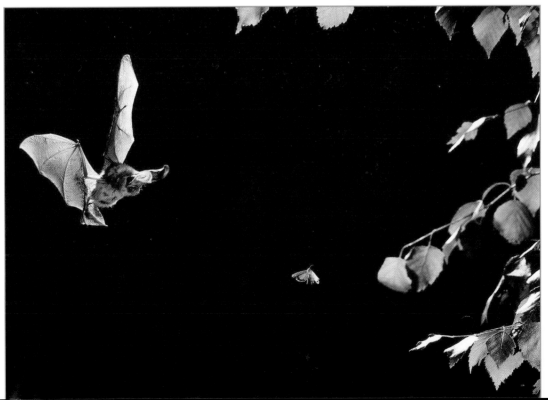

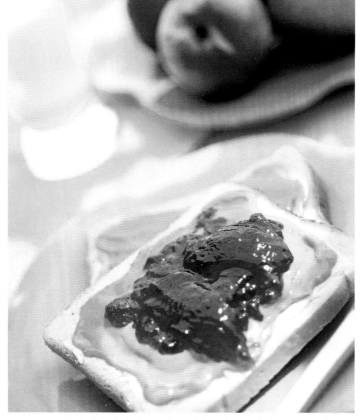

Do you think this is a healthy breakfast? Why?
What do you like to eat for breakfast?

What happens if you skip breakfast? You'll have just enough energy to breathe, pump blood, and move your muscles. You won't have the nutrients to think well in school, or do your best in sports, or grow.

Great breakfasts have foods from the fruit group, the bread group, and the protein group for strength and growth and brain power. The meal could be as simple as a bowl of cereal, a glass of juice, and some raisins on the way to the bus, but break that fast!

Bats rest after their breakfast, then hunt again later at night. You eat in spurts, too, at breakfast, lunch, and dinner.

Except for when you eat breakfast, it doesn't matter what time your body gets its nutrients. And some food servings can be eaten as snacks to keep energy levels high between meals.

What food groups are represented in this refrigerator?

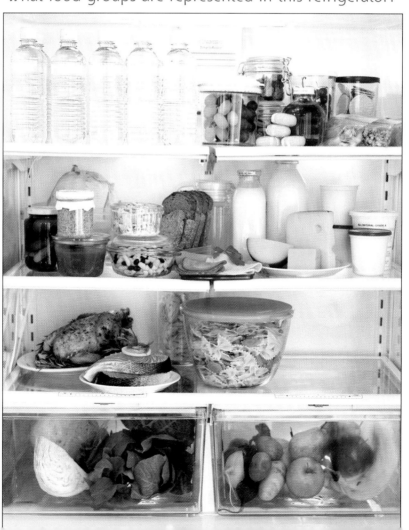

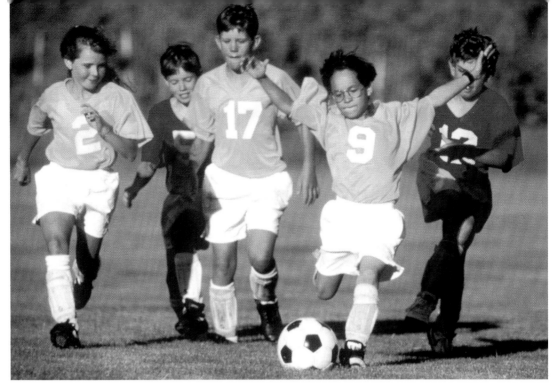

If you play this hard for 90 minutes or if it is very hot outside, you may need to replace the salt you lose as you sweat, as well as the calories you burn.

Your nutrient needs change for high-energy athletic events. Athletes start the day with a good breakfast. A few hours before the game, they eat extra servings from the bread group for lasting energy.

While they play, athletes get quick energy from oranges or other fruits and juices instead of sugary snacks. Afterward, they eat more fruit or sandwiches to replace the calories they've burned.

The next day, athletes go back to eating meals and snacks the regular food-pyramid way!

Clues from a Camel

Camels can live for 17 days without taking a drink of water. You couldn't last more than a few days without this special nutrient.

How does the camel survive so well on its long desert journeys? One reason is that the camel doesn't sweat and lose water unless its body temperature gets very high. If you took a walk in a desert, it wouldn't take long before you became overheated and started to sweat.

Camels can travel 80 miles (129 kilometers) in a day without stopping for water. You could do the same—but you'd need to be in a speeding car!

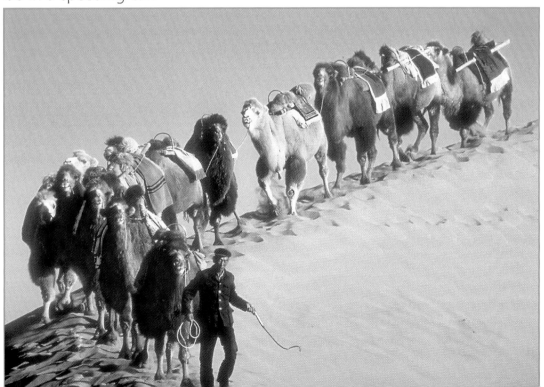

You need water! This important nutrient keeps your whole body running smoothly. A 60-pound (27-kilogram) child needs four full glasses of water (or other fluids like juice or milk) every day. Bigger kids need more. If you are exercising, you need much more. Why?

The reason is that you lose water with every breath. The harder and faster you breathe, the more water vapor you lose. As you sweat to keep your body cool, you're losing even more water.

A marathon is only a little more than 26 miles (41.8 kilometers) long, but runners need to drink water before, during, and after the event.

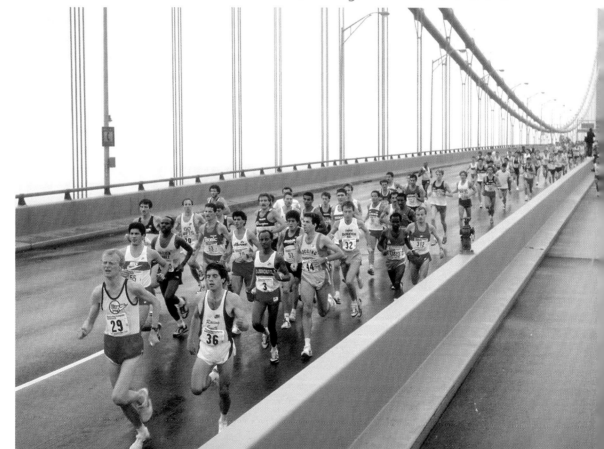

The same thing happens on hot sunny days. You sweat and you keep losing water—and salt. If the amount of water in your body drops too low, you can get **dehydrated**. Being dehydrated can cause

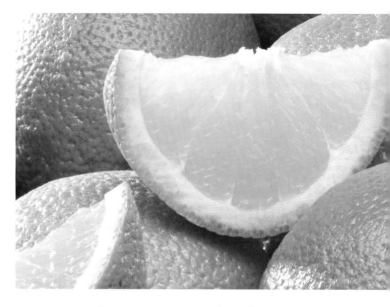

a headache, then muscle cramps, then a stomachache. You need water to keep from getting sick!

Anything wet enough to drink has water in it. So do juicy fruits like oranges, pineapples, grapes, berries, and, of course, watermelons. Or you can just drink plain water.

Make Your Own Sports Drink

1 quart of 100% fruit juice (your favorite kind)
1 cup of water
3/4 teaspoon of salt

1. Mix the juice and water in a large pitcher.
2. Add the salt.
3. Keep chilled.

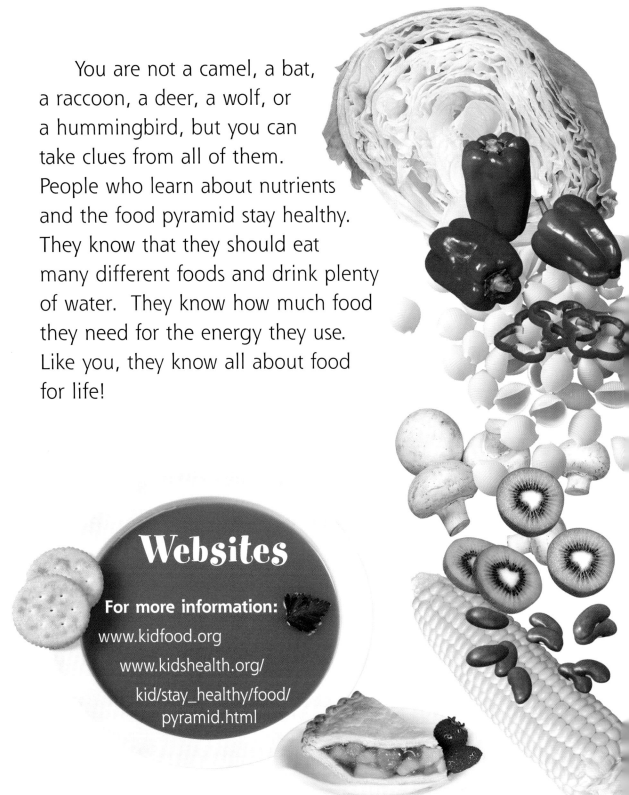

You are not a camel, a bat, a raccoon, a deer, a wolf, or a hummingbird, but you can take clues from all of them. People who learn about nutrients and the food pyramid stay healthy. They know that they should eat many different foods and drink plenty of water. They know how much food they need for the energy they use. Like you, they know all about food for life!

Websites

For more information:
www.kidfood.org
www.kidshealth.org/
kid/stay_healthy/food/
pyramid.html

Glossary

calorie: a unit scientists use to measure the energy stored in food

carbohydrate: a nutrient found in plants that is a major energy source for people and animals. Carbohydrates are found in foods such as bread, cereal, potatoes, and pasta.

carnivore: an animal that eats mainly meat

dehydrate: to reduce the amount of water in something

diet: what a person usually eats and drinks

digest: to break down food so it can be used by the body

fast: to not eat

herbivore: an animal that eats mainly plants

mineral: a natural substance that is neither animal nor plant and that usually comes from the ground. Minerals such as iron, calcium, copper, and zinc help keep the body strong.

nutrient: a substance in food that is necessary for good health. Proteins, carbohydrates, vitamins, and minerals are all nutrients.

omnivore: an animal that eats both plants and animals

protein: a chemical substance made by plants and animals that is necessary for growth and for keeping the body strong. Meat, chicken, fish, and dairy foods contain lots of protein.

vitamin: a natural substance made by plants and animals that is necessary in small amounts to the nutrition of most animals

Index